HOME
REMEDIES

BRONCHITIS, ALLERGIES, COLD & FLU

CONTENTS

Publications International, Ltd.

ALLERGIES

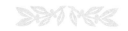

Allergies occur when your immune system goes overboard in its defense of your body, reacting to harmless visitors as if they were alien invaders bent on destruction. This out-of-proportion response can leave you miserable. But you can take steps to temper such overreactions and ease the discomfort of allergy symptoms.

Your immune system is your own personal bodyguard—constantly on the lookout for any intruders it considers harmful, such as illness-causing viruses and bacteria. When it detects such a trespasser, the immune system marshals its forces to battle the interloper and flush out, kill, or neutralize it. In this way, it helps to keep you healthy. If you have allergies, however, your immune system has difficulty distinguishing the bad guys from innocent bystanders. Like a nervous rookie, it sees danger everywhere and tends to overreact, responding with too much force against substances—like dust and pollen—that won't do you any actual harm. Those harmless substances are called allergens.

Roughly 1 in 5—or 50 million—Americans suffer from some type of allergy, of which there are many. The list of substances capable of triggering an allergic reaction is even longer. Among the most common are:

- Pollen from trees, grasses, and weeds, which is responsible for hay fever and other seasonal allergies

- Dust, which typically contains dust mites and their droppings (potent allergens on their own), additional animal allergens, bits of fabric, bacteria, and other debris

- Molds, which can thrive in moist environments both indoors and out

- Animal dander—flakes of dead skin from cats, dogs, or rodents that carry allergenic proteins from the animal's sweat and saliva

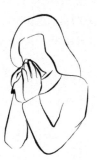

- Cockroaches

- Medications

- Foods

- Poisonous plants, such as poison ivy, oak, or sumac

- Latex

- Insect bites and stings

The body's first lines of defense against invaders include the eyes, nose, mouth, lungs, skin, and stomach. They are the most common places for the body to encounter a foreign substance. So when a hyperactive immune system reacts to an allergen, it sets off an inflammatory response in one or more of these battleground body parts. Symptoms of the battle may occur individually or in combination, can range from barely noticeable to incapacitating, and often depend on how the allergen is contacted. For example, if you inhale an allergen, you may experience nasal congestion; sneezing; a runny nose; itching in your nose, ears, or throat; postnasal drip; and possibly a cough. You may also have a headache due to sinus pressure, and your throat may feel a bit raw from your attempts to clear postnasal drip. If the allergen gets in your eyes, they may become itchy, watery, swollen, and red. If you have a skin allergy, contact with the allergen may cause a red rash or hives, itchiness in the area of contact, and possibly blisters and peeling. Use of a medication to which you are allergic can produce symptoms throughout the body. If you have a food allergy and inadvertently eat the offending food, you may experience itching in your mouth, throat, or nose; stomach cramps; nausea and vomiting; diarrhea; or, in severe cases, a life-threatening reaction called anaphylaxis. People who are extremely allergic to insect venom can also develop anaphylaxis after a bite or sting.

The symptoms of anaphylaxis may include wheezing; widespread hives; swelling of the face, eyes, throat, lips, and/or tongue; shortness of breath; tightness in the throat or chest; difficulty breathing; low blood pressure; dizziness; loss of consciousness; and even death. An anaphylactic reaction can progress quickly, so medical treatment should be sought at the first sign of this condition.

In many cases, however, allergy symptoms are difficult to differentiate from the symptoms of other disorders and illnesses, such as a cold or the flu, a problem with nasal anatomy, or a food intolerance. To rule out other possible causes and help you avoid the use of inappropriate remedies, have your allergies properly diagnosed by a board-certified allergist. And if you have ever suffered a severe allergic reaction, working with an allergist is an absolute must.

The remedies and strategies that follow are designed to ease allergy symptoms and reduce your exposure to common allergens; they may be used alone or in combination with over-the-counter medications and/or therapies prescribed by your allergist.

SOOTHE YOUR SYMPTOMS

To ease the discomfort of an allergy attack:

- Most allergy symptoms disappear soon after exposure ends, so the best treatment is to get away from the trigger as soon as you can. If cats make you sneeze or itch, for example, and you've just stepped into a household with cats, make the visit as short as possible. Don't touch or pick up the animal or let it climb on or rub up against you. Also avoid touching your eyes or nose, and be sure to wash your hands when you leave.

- If exposure to pollen or dander has made your eyes itchy and irritated, first wash your hands and then rinse your eyes with cool, clean water. The coolness will be soothing, and rinsing should help wash away allergens.

- Motor-vehicle exhaust can worsen an allergic reaction, so avoid walking along traffic-congested roads when you're suffering respiratory allergy symptoms.

- Leave allergens at the door. When time outdoors triggers seasonal allergy symptoms, take steps to keep the outdoors from following you into your home. (This same advice applies if you have a pet allergy and have just spent time

SKIN ALLERGY RELIEF

If contact with an allergen has produced an itchy skin rash, try the itch-relief remedies in the "Poison Ivy, Oak & Sumac" profile in the booklet *Home Remedies: First Aid for Small Emergencies*.

in a cat or dog household.) Leave your shoes at the door and remove the clothes you were wearing when exposed, because they likely picked up allergens. Then take a shower or at least rinse your hair and wash your hands and face; sticky yellow pollen or other airborne allergens that have collected on your skin and in your hair and eyebrows can easily end up in your eyes, nose, or airways, where they will continue to fuel your allergy misery.

- If your allergy is causing sinus congestion that's giving you a headache or pain around your eyes and nose, avoid lying flat; it will only increase the pressure and pain. Instead, keep your head and shoulders propped up at an angle by tucking extra pillows between your upper body and the mattress or between the mattress and box spring.

- Apply moist heat to help lessen discomfort caused by stuffed sinuses. If your sinuses feel like they're about to explode and take your eyeballs with them, you can get quick relief by stepping into a hot shower and directing the water at your face. If you can't take a shower, soak a washcloth in very warm water, sit down, lean back slightly, and place the washcloth over your nose and upper-cheek area for a few minutes. The moist heat should encourage the sinuses to drain, helping to relieve the uncomfortable pressure. Rewarm the washcloth as needed.

- To ease nasal allergy symptoms, use saline (saltwater) solution to rinse allergens and inflammatory cells from your nasal passages. Ready-made saline solution is available at drugstores, as are kits containing teapot-like vessels— called neti pots—designed specifically for flushing out the nasal passages. But you can make your own fresh saline solution daily by boiling a pint of water for 2 minutes, letting it cool, and mixing in a teaspoon of salt and a pinch of baking soda. (Distilled water can be used in place of the boiled water.) Then, while standing over a sink or bowl, squirt the solution into one nostril at a time using a bulb syringe and let it drain back out through your nose or down your throat and out through your mouth. Do this once or twice daily. But if you have asthma, check with your doctor before trying this remedy.

- Drink plenty of water. If you don't stay well hydrated, your nasal secretions and mucus will become thicker and more difficult to clear.

- Savor a cup of hot green tea with lemon 2 or 3 times daily. Hot tea with lemon is astringent and helps cut through phlegm and break up congestion due to allergies. And some research suggests that green tea specifically is rich in an antioxidant that may discourage your immune system from setting off all those allergy symptoms in response to harmless substances. Adding a little honey to the tea will soothe a raw throat. In between sips, lean over your tea so the steam can help unplug your head.

- Skip milk when allergies act up. Dairy thickens mucus.

- Enjoy a spicy dish that includes onion, garlic, cayenne pepper, fenugreek, or hot ginger; it'll help chase out congestion by thinning mucus.

- Get more omega-3s. These healthy fatty acids—found naturally and in abundance in fatty fish, such as salmon—help fight inflammation, including the kinds of inflammation that occur in an allergic reaction. So when you're struggling with allergy symptoms, try including omega-3-rich fish in your diet a few times a week.

- Try to rest and relax more when your allergies flare up. Getting too little sleep and downtime increases stress, which in turn appears to increase inflammation and spur more intense allergy symptoms, according to research.

OUTSMART ALLERGENS

The most basic and effective way to control allergies is to avoid the allergens as much as possible. The following remedies can minimize exposure to common allergens:

- If you suffer seasonal allergies or if outdoor air pollutants trigger or aggravate your allergies, monitor weather reports for your area daily. Many weather-information outlets provide alerts when conditions in your area are likely to result in high concentrations of various pollens, molds, ozone, and other air pollutants. On those days, spend as little time outdoors as possible, and if you typically exercise outside, move your workout indoors.

- When you go outdoors during allergy season—especially on warm, dry, and/or windy days—wear sunglasses, your regular prescription eyeglasses, or even a pair of glasses with plano lenses to help keep pollen out of your eyes. And if you need to be outdoors for more than a few minutes when pollen or mold counts are especially high, consider wearing a dust mask over your nose and mouth.

- Kick smoke out of your home. Tobacco smoke—whether first- or secondhand—can trigger or aggravate an allergy attack. Away from home, avoid smoky rooms or standing near anyone who is smoking—even outdoors. And, of course, if you still light up, stop it!

IS IT A FOOD ALLERGY?

Do you feel congested after you eat dairy products? Does red meat make you sluggish? Does sugar give you a headache? If you answered "yes" to any of these questions, you probably *don't* have a food allergy.

Many people confuse food allergies with food intolerances. A person who has a food intolerance may be able to handle small amounts of the problem food without experiencing symptoms, but those who have a true food allergy must avoid even tiny traces of the allergenic food. And while food intolerance can trigger unpleasant symptoms like those mentioned above, a true food allergy can be extremely serious—even deadly.

If you are allergic to a food, the reaction will be almost immediate; within a few minutes to 2 hours of eating it, symptoms will develop. The most common are itching in the mouth; hives; diffuse swelling around the eyes and mouth; nasal congestion, sneezing, or breathing difficulties; dizziness; and nausea, vomiting, diarrhea, or abdominal cramps. In severe cases, extremely low blood pressure, swelling or constriction of the throat or airways, or loss of consciousness may occur. In these instances, emergency medical attention is required.

- Keep the windows of your home and auto shut at all times to keep pollen and outdoor molds from blowing in. If it's an option, set the ventilation system in your car to "recirculate," so pollen-carrying outside air is not constantly introduced into the vehicle.

- Expose what lies below. Carpets are notorious for harboring dust mites—microscopic bugs that feed on the dead skin cells we constantly shed and whose corpses and drop-pings spark allergy symptoms in millions of people. Bare floors, vacuumed and damp-mopped frequently, will help keep your home's dust-mite population down (you can't get rid of them all). If you can't remove all the carpeting in your home, at least go with bare floors in your bedroom; studies show the bedroom has more dust mites than any other room in the home, and you probably spend about a third of your time there every day. If you find totally bare floors in the bedroom too cold, use small throw rugs that you launder frequently.

- Any carpeting you can't remove must be kept as clean as possible. It should be vacuumed at least twice a week. Just be aware that many vacuums blow small particles of dust back into the air. To help minimize this problem, use a vacuum with a HEPA filter, and follow the manufacturer's recommendations for cleaning or replacing the filter.

- Control household dust wisely. Cleaning the surfaces in your home at least once a week can go far in helping to control allergy symptoms that are triggered or aggravated by dust. But if done improperly, dusting may actually make things worse. Your aim is to remove dust, not just spread it around or send it into the air. To do that, avoid feather dusters and other dry-dusting methods, which scatter rather than contain dust. You may also need to avoid commercial cleaners and dusting sprays, which often contain fragrances or other ingredients that can trigger or increase allergy symptoms. Instead, try:

  - Dusting wood furniture with a soft, clean cloth damp-ened with a mixture of 1 part lemon juice to 2 parts vegetable oil.

- Cleaning floors (wood or otherwise) with a mop moistened with vinegar.

- Wiping down most other common household surfaces with a cloth and a hypoallergenic cleaning solution you can make at home by combining 2 cups hot water, 1 small squirt of dishwashing liquid, 1 teaspoon baking soda, 1 teaspoon borax, and about 2 teaspoons distilled vinegar in a clean spray bottle.

- If dusting even with hypoallergenic cleaners seems to fuel your allergy symptoms, however, you may simply need to ask another household member to dust (perhaps you can do the dishes or laundry instead) or hire a cleaning service.

- If you're allergic to dust mites, keep fabric-covered furniture to a minimum. Wood, leather, and vinyl furniture—which can be damp-dusted—are better choices.

- Choose washable curtains over venetian blinds so you can regularly wash away dust mites hiding in the fabric. The slats of blinds are notorious dust collectors. If you can't replace all the blinds in your home, be sure to vacuum or dust them well during your thorough weekly cleaning.

- Encase pillows and mattresses in airtight plastic or vinyl covers that are impermeable to allergens. Otherwise you'll be laying your head in a virtual garden of dust mites every time you hit the sack. These covers are usually available online or at department stores and bedding outlets.

- Even with allergen-impermeable pillow and mattress covers in place, you should wash your sheets, pillowcases, and comforter every 7 to 10 days in sudsy water as hot as they'll tolerate. (It takes hot water to kill dust mites.) Wash your mattress pad and synthetic blankets every 2 weeks.

• Try not to keep anything in your bedroom that doesn't have to be there. Stuffed animals, perfume bottles, books and magazines, picture frames, knickknacks, and such tend to collect dust and will only contribute to your allergy misery. If you don't have any other space to store such items, seal bulky items in covered plastic tubs that you dust at least once a week, and display pictures and knickknacks in a closed glass-front cabinet that you wipe down regularly as well.

• Track the humidity level in your home using a device called a hygrometer, available at hardware stores. Dust mites love a humid environment, which allows them to reproduce like crazy. Mold, too, is a denizen of damp places. To help keep these allergens in check, therefore, aim to keep the humidity level in your home in the range of 30 to 50 percent. If the hygrometer shows the humidity level is above 60 percent, run a dehumidifier or an air conditioner; either will pull moisture from the air. (Carefully follow the manufacturer's instructions for cleaning and maintaining your dehumidifier or air conditioner.) In addition, run the exhaust fan in the kitchen when the stove or oven is in use, and run the exhaust fan in the bathroom whenever anyone is bathing to help keep household humidity levels in the allergy-wise range.

• Don't cut the grass. During pollen season, a grass-allergic person is better off letting someone else—anyone else—mow the lawn. Call your local county extension service and find out when the pollination season occurs in your area, then arrange for a lawn-care company, friend, or relative to cut your grass during that time. (As a rule, in many parts of the country, people who are allergic to grass should avoid mowing between May and early July.)

HELLO, DOCTOR?

If your allergies make you cough and wheeze and make it hard for you to breathe freely, see an allergist. You may have allergic asthma, which should be monitored by a doctor. People with allergic asthma, which is sometimes mistaken for bronchitis, often need prescription medications and should not attempt home remedies for symptom relief without their doctor's approval.

- If you own a dog or cat but are allergic to its dander—and can't imagine finding a new home for your furry friend—bathe your pet frequently (or have someone do it for you). Dogs and cats constantly shed dead skin cells called dander, which is a common allergen. Fortunately, this allergen dissolves in water, so regular warm baths—without soap—can help rinse away some of the problem. If you start bathing your cat or dog early in its life, chances are higher that bath time will become a harmonious experience for both of you. Bathe your pet every other week, and always wash your hands right after you've had direct contact with your little buddy.

- If you are allergic to the dander from your cat or dog, keep your pet out of your bedroom, even if the pet is bathed regularly.

- When planning a trip, call ahead to find a room that will be easier on your allergies. Ask for a nonsmoking room that's not on the lower level, since a ground-floor room may have been flooded in the past and may still harbor mold. Choose a place that doesn't allow pets. And if possible, bring your own vinyl- or plastic-encased pillow.

BRONCHITIS

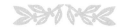

When a cold or another upper respiratory
infection seems to be fading but instead
morphs into a harsh phlegmy cough that
makes you sound like a harbor seal,
you've probably developed bronchitis.
As your body fights this storm in your chest,
some simple home remedies can make
the battle less bruising.

ACUTE BRONCHITIS

Bronchitis is an inflammation of the bronchial tubes, the
oxygen passageways in your lungs. It comes in a very common acute (short-term) version, which usually goes away
on its own, and a chronic (long-term) and far more serious version that is considered a chronic obstructive pul-
monary disease (COPD). Acute bronchitis is an infection
of the bronchial tubes that's most often caused by a virus,
frequently the same one that causes colds, although the flu
virus is a common culprit as well. (While acute bronchitis
can also be caused by bacteria or even fungi, they are only
rarely to blame.) Acute bronchitis often develops on the
heels of a cold or the flu, when the body's resistance is down
and the lungs may already be slightly irritated. Likewise,
anyone whose resistance is low or who has another type of
chronic lung irritation or injury—especially from exposure

to cigarette smoke or other toxic gases—is at increased risk of developing bronchitis.

The viruses that cause bronchitis can be passed to other folks the same way cold and flu viruses are: An infected person coughs, spraying viral particles either into the air, where they can be breathed in by others, or onto their own hands, from where they can be transferred to common objects (like doorknobs, glasses, and pens) or to other people by a handshake. Once a person gets the virus on their hands, they can easily infect themselves by simply touching their own eyes, nose, or mouth.

The virus attacks the inner walls of the bronchial tubes, which then swell and produce greatly increased amounts of thick, often yellow or green mucus. (The airways normally produce about an ounce a day of thin clear or white mucus, which helps trap and remove foreign particles.) The lung irritation and mucus trigger a throaty, persistent, productive hacking—the hallmark of acute bronchitis. It can be accompanied by an irritated throat (from coughing), burning or aching beneath the breastbone, tightness in the chest, wheezing or shortness of breath, and/or a "rattling" sensation in the lungs or chest. A low-grade fever, chills, and achiness may also occur. The irritation caused by the virus also leaves the respiratory tract vulnerable to other complications, such as pneumonia.

If you have an underlying chronic disease or suffer from asthma, allergies, COPD, or any other serious respiratory or heart problem, you need to contact your doctor if you develop symptoms of acute bronchitis. Bronchitis symptoms in infants, the elderly, or anyone with a weak immune system also require medical attention. If you're otherwise healthy, however, you will likely have to allow the infection to simply run its course. Antibiotics, after all, are useless against viral infections. Fortunately, acute bronchitis generally goes away on its own within a few days to two weeks, although the cough can sometimes linger for weeks or even months. Until your body has shaken the infection, there are some things you can do to decrease discomfort and help your body heal:

- Take in extra liquids. It will help keep mucus, or sputum, more fluid and therefore easier to cough up. And that's a good thing, because coughing is your body's way of expelling the extra mucus it produces to trap and remove irritants and invaders from your lungs. (Using an over-the-counter cough suppressant on a productive cough—one that brings up mucus—actually works against your body's healing efforts.) Decaffeinated liquids are best, since caffeine can have a slight dehydrating effect. Some people find warm liquids, such as soup and hot decaffeinated or herbal tea, more soothing on a throat that's raw from coughing and clearing; others find that cold liquids, like fruit juices and ice water, feel better.

- Try some bay leaf tea. This age-old home remedy acts as an expectorant, encouraging your lungs to cough out the excess mucus that's interfering with your breathing. To make the tea, tear a fresh or dried bay leaf into pieces, steep in 1 cup boiling water for 5 to 10 minutes, strain, and drink up to 3 cups throughout the day.

- Gargle with warm salt water. Gargling with salt water may provide a double dose of relief by soothing your raw

WATCH FOR COMPLICATIONS

While letting nature take its course is generally the best treatment for acute bronchitis, complications can occur, so stay alert for signs that it's time to see your doctor. The most worrisome complications include pneumonia, sinus infection, and ear infection, which may need to be treated with prescription medications. Signs that complications may be developing include a persistent high fever (not typical with bronchitis), severe shortness of breath, prolonged coughing spells or a cough that lasts more than 4 to 6 weeks, severe chest pain, pain behind the eyes, or ear pain. Also be on the lookout for blood in your sputum or sputum that changes dramatically in color or consistency, and report it to your doctor. In addition, tell your doctor if you suffer frequent bouts of bronchitis, since this may indicate that you have a more serious underlying respiratory problem.

throat and cutting through some of the mucus that has you repeatedly clearing your throat. It only takes 1 teaspoon of salt in a glass (8 to 10 ounces) of warm water; too much salt can make your throat burn, and too little will be ineffective. Gargle as often as needed, but spit the salty water out afterward.

- Another good way to help clear mucus and soothe a mild sore throat is to drink hot lemon-spiked water. To prepare it, either grate 1 teaspoon lemon rind into 1 cup boiling water and steep 5 minutes or add a lemon wedge to a pot containing 1 cup water, bring to a boil, remove from the heat, and let steep 5 minutes before straining out the lemon and drinking.

- Inhale warm, moist air to help break up mucus and ease coughing. If you're having a coughing fit, try standing in a steamy shower with the bathroom door closed. Or set a pot of heated water on a trivet or pot holder placed on a table, drape a towel over your head, lean your face over the pot, and inhale the steam. You might also consider investing in a warm-mist humidifier for your bedroom, since you spend so much of every day in there; just be aware that you will need to be diligent about following the manufacturer's instructions for daily and weekly cleaning of the machine in order to prevent the growth of mold. If you have allergies or asthma, consult your doctor before using a humidifier.

- Use eucalyptus. Eucalyptus oil—applied topically or inhaled—has long been used to help treat nose and chest congestion, including the buildup of excess mucus in the lungs that occurs in acute bronchitis. You can find it in various over-the-counter rubs, which you can smear on your chest, as directed on the package, to help loosen phlegm. You may also be able to find products that exude eucalyptus vapors when mixed into a hot bath or added to a vaporizer. But you can also create your own eucalyptus treatments for bronchitis using eucalyptus oil purchased from a health food retailer. For a topical treatment that you can rub on your congested chest, add 15 to 30 drops eucalyptus oil to a carrier such as olive oil or sesame oil. For a tabletop steam treatment that includes a eucalyptus kick, add 6 to 10 drops eucalyptus oil to every 2 cups boiling water before following the rest of the instructions in the preceding remedy.

- Eat more C-rich foods. Research suggests that getting more vitamin C may speed recovery from acute bronchitis. The vitamin is found abundantly in a variety of fruits and vegetables, including oranges, bell peppers, strawberries, broccoli, and cantaloupe.

- Rest, rest, and rest some more. Trying to keep up your regular routine while you have acute bronchitis will likely make you feel more run-down and hinder your body's ability to fight the infection.

- Take aspirin or ibuprofen to relieve pain in the chest muscles. If a bout with bronchitis produces muscle pain in the chest, these anti-inflammatory pain medications may provide some relief. Acetaminophen also eases pain but does not have an anti-inflammatory effect and so may be less helpful. (Because of the risk of a potentially deadly reaction called Reye's syndrome, don't give aspirin to children unless specifically directed to do so by their doctor; use acetaminophen instead.)

- Use over-the-counter cough medicine only if you must. The best cough medicines for acute bronchitis contain the expectorant guaifenesin, which helps the lungs get rid of mucus. But if you can't bear another minute of hacking—especially if coughing has been preventing you from getting the sleep your body needs to recover—you can try a medicine that contains the cough suppressant dextromethorphan. Be sure to read and follow the package instructions, and take it only as often as necessary. Combination products should generally be avoided; decongestants, antihistamines, and alcohol (all common ingredients in combination products sold as treatments for colds, flu, allergies, sinus troubles, congestion, and the like) have no role in the treatment of coughs and may even increase discomfort by causing side effects. Most candy-type cough drops act only as demulcents on the throat—in other words, their soothing properties are due largely to their sugar content. A little honey—alone or dissolved into hot tea with lemon—is likely to be just as beneficial.

CHRONIC BRONCHITIS

Unlike acute bronchitis, which usually hangs around for just a few days, chronic bronchitis doesn't know when to leave. In fact, this inflammation of the bronchial tubes may become permanent or keep coming back like a boomerang. Bronchitis is diagnosed as chronic when a person coughs up mucus for 3 straight months or more, 2 years in a row.

Chronic bronchitis is the result of continued irritation of the airways, from substances such as air pollution and cigarette smoke—including secondhand smoke. Indeed, cigarette smoking is the primary cause of the disease.

Symptoms of chronic bronchitis include:

- Smoker's cough—a recurring morning cough that brings up mucus

- Shortness of breath, especially after the disease has progressed

- Wheezing and coughing that are nearly continuous in the disease's final stages

There is no cure for chronic bronchitis, although removing the cause of the irritation can lessen symptoms. (For smokers who develop symptoms of the disease, quitting is essential.) Chronic bronchitis usually leads to other respiratory diseases such as emphysema and pneumonia. In some cases, it is fatal. Because of its seriousness, a person with chronic bronchitis needs to be under a physician's care.

In conjunction with a physician's prescribed treatments and instructions, the following measures may make breathing a little easier:

- Get flu and pneumonia shots every year. Those with chronic bronchitis are highly susceptible to these illnesses,

BRONCHITIS AND SMOKERS

Smoking is a habit that is continually under fire for its negative impact on a person's health. And rightly so. It has been proven to be a significant contributing factor in emphysema, lung cancer, heart disease, and several other serious illnesses. It leaves you more vulnerable to acute bronchitis and other respiratory infections, aggravates any such infection that does take hold, and slows your body's ability to heal. Because a smoker's bronchial tubes are already irritated, any additional inflammation caused by acute bronchitis may require medical attention. Smoking is also the primary cause of chronic bronchitis. Needless to say, refraining from smoking—or at least cutting way back—is essential when battling a case of acute bronchitis. To treat or prevent chronic bronchitis, quitting for good and avoiding exposure to other people's cigarette smoke are essential.

and these illnesses are far more dangerous for people with chronic bronchitis.

- In addition to quitting smoking, chronic bronchitis sufferers should avoid smoky environments and stay inside whenever air pollution levels are high. Such information can typically be found on daily TV, radio, or online weather reports for your locality.

- Exercise your lungs. Regular moderate physical activity—such as brisk walking or swimming—can strengthen your lungs and make breathing easier. Playing a wind instrument, such as a clarinet or saxophone, can also enhance your lung capacity. Just avoid pushing yourself too hard—your doctor and perhaps a physical therapist can help you determine the type, amount, and intensity level of exercise that's appropriate. And be sure to move your workout indoors on high-pollution days.

- Give your immune system plenty of ammunition. The vitamin C (along with other beneficial nutrients) provided by many fruits and vegetables can help to keep your immune system strong and protect your vulnerable lungs from potentially serious infections. Citrus fruits are excellent sources of this vitamin, as are broccoli, cauliflower, brussels sprouts, bell peppers, papaya, cantaloupe, pineapple, and strawberries.

- When bronchitis symptoms flare, go easy on dairy products, sugar, and chocolate. They promote the secretion of mucus, which will only aggravate the symptoms you are already experiencing.

COLD & FLU

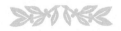

We should probably add "common cold" and "flu" to "death" and "taxes" on the list of things we can't escape in life. For most of us, fortunately, these viral infections are short-lived and harmless. And while medicine can't cure them, home remedies can make them easier to endure.

THE COMMON COLD

More than 200 viruses are capable of causing colds. When you catch a cold, virus particles attach to cells in the mucous membranes lining the inside of your nose and throat. Like aliens in a sci-fi movie, they punch holes in the cell membranes and inject viral genetic material, turning your own cells into tiny virus-making factories.

In response, your body defends itself: Your nose and throat release chemicals that mobilize the immune system; injured cells produce chemicals that trigger inflammation and attract infection-fighting white blood cells; tiny blood vessels widen, allowing plasma (blood fluid) and more white blood cells to enter the infected area; your body temperature rises slightly, enhancing the immune response; and histamine is released, increasing the production of nasal mucus in an effort to trap viral particles and remove them from the body.

The symptoms you experience as a cold—sneezing, stuffy nose, watery eyes, sore throat, cough, mild headache or muscle aches, and perhaps a touch of fever—are actually part of your body's natural immune response. And by the time these symptoms appear, the virus has already been attacking your body—and making you capable of infecting others—for probably 24 to 36 hours.

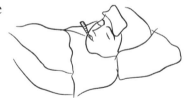

INFLUENZA AKA "THE FLU"

The word "flu" has become a catch-all term for any affliction of the upper respiratory tract, and it is often also improperly used in the term "stomach flu" to denote infections of the gastrointestinal tract. But the condition it actually refers to—influenza—is a specific viral respiratory infection that strikes every year, typically between October and April.

While there are two major strains of the flu virus—influenza A and influenza B—each strain constantly undergoes slight changes, so getting the flu one year doesn't guarantee protection against the following year's flu bug. (That's also why flu shots aren't always effective in preventing influenza.)

An influenza virus is spread much like a cold virus; you can get it either by inhaling an airborne droplet from an infected person's cough or sneeze or by touching something (doorknob, computer keyboard, phone, eating utensils, etc.) that has an influenza virus on it. (The virus can live for several hours on inanimate objects.) And because infected people are contagious for a day or two before showing symptoms, many carriers don't know they're spreading the virus.

Regardless of the strain, the symptoms are generally the same and develop within 72 hours of exposure to the virus.

INFLUENZA MYTHS

There are a few myths about the flu that continue to prevail despite evidence that disproves them. One is what folks often refer to as the "24-hour flu" or "stomach flu." This illness is marked by the sudden onset of vomiting and diarrhea and a general feeling of malaise. It can be quite intense in the first few hours but tends to subside completely after 24 hours. While this illness is indeed caused by a virus, it's not caused by the influenza virus and therefore is not a flu at all. The correct term for this type of upset is "gastroenteritis," which indicates an inflammation of the digestive tract.

Another common myth about influenza is that being cold or chilled makes us more susceptible to it. Several scientific studies on humans have shown that those exposed to temperature extremes for several hours are no more likely to get the flu than are those kept comfortably warm and dry. Severe chills are indeed an early symptom of flu, and this may lead people to believe they "caught a chill" that somehow led to their illness.

One more common myth is that using medicine to keep the fever down helps us get over the illness. Although you may feel a bit better after taking something to lower your fever, you may also be extending your bout with the flu. Animal studies suggest that it takes the body longer to eradicate the flu virus if its core temperature is lowered with medication.

Although the symptoms can mimic a bad cold, there are some definite differences. Classic signs of the flu include those notorious muscle aches, a fever that usually ranges from 101°F to 103°F in adults (higher in children), chills, a dry cough, and extreme fatigue. These symptoms accompany coldlike problems such as a runny and stuffy nose, headache, and sore throat. Nausea and vomiting may also occur.

It typically takes 7 to 10 days to fully recover from the flu. Since the flu can lead to more serious illnesses, like pneumonia, tell your physician if any symptoms worsen after you start feeling better.

DO-IT-YOURSELF RELIEF

You can't beg, steal, borrow, or buy a cure for either the cold or the flu, but you can use the following home remedies to ease your discomfort and help your body rid itself of the viral invaders as quickly as possible:

- Give your immune system a hand by getting extra rest and sleep, especially early on when symptoms are at their worst. Your body has its hands full battling the cold or flu virus. Don't make it split its energy and resources between defending your health and doing work, chores, or other activities that don't need to be done immediately.

- Even if you exercise regularly, don't force yourself to work out. If you're in the grips of the flu bug, you're probably so fatigued and achy that lifting your head off the pillow is all the workout you can manage anyhow. But even if you only have a cold, you should probably skip exercising for at least a day or two when your symptoms are at their worst. Once your symptoms start to fade, however, a little movement may actually be beneficial. Indeed, when they're recovering from colds, many regular exercisers report easier breathing and other symptom improvement after engaging in light physical activity. Still, it's important to listen to your body and let it tell you whether it's time to start getting back into the swing of physical activity.

WORTH REMEMBERING

Every now and then, a new influenza virus emerges that causes an unusually high number of infections and deaths across a wide area. The last such "pandemic" struck the United States in 2009.

- Stay warm. Cold air and drafts don't cause colds or the flu, of course, but you're likely to feel more comfortable if you stay indoors and covered, especially if you have a fever. Forcing your body to work harder to keep you warm will rob it of energy it could better use fighting the infection.

- If a fever has you feeling miserable, get some relief from ginger tea. It will make you sweat, which will help cool your body and make you feel more comfortable. Thinly slice a piece of fresh gingerroot that's about the size of your thumb. Put the ginger slices and 4 cups water into a pot and bring to a boil. Reduce heat, cover, and simmer for about 30 minutes. Remove the pot from the heat and let cool for a half hour. Strain out the ginger slices, pour yourself 1 cup, add a little honey to taste, and sip. Repeat 3 more times throughout the day.

- Stop smoking. You'll feel better sooner and cut your risk of getting even sicker. Doctors say smokers have a tougher time shaking off a cold than nonsmokers do. Worse, smoking while you have a cold or flu irritates the bronchial tubes, which increases the risk of developing pneumonia and other complications. Smoking also depresses the immune system.

WHEN TO CALL THE DOCTOR

While most colds can be effectively treated at home, call your doctor if:

- You have a headache and stiff neck with no other cold symptoms

- You have a headache and sore throat with no other cold symptoms

- You have cold symptoms and significant pain across your nose and face that doesn't go away

- You have a fever above 101°F (adults) that lasts more than 3 days

- Your infant develops a rectal temperature of 100.2°F or higher

- Your child develops a rectal temperature of 102°F or higher

- Your cold symptoms seem to be going away, but you suddenly develop a fever

- You have a "dry" cough—one that doesn't bring up phlegm—for more than 10 days

- You cough up blood or your cough is accompanied by severe chest pain or shortness of breath

- Drink plenty of fluids to keep virus-trapping mucus flowing freely, so it's easier to expel. Drink at least 8 ounces of water and other decaffeinated liquids every 2 hours.

- Fill some of your fluid needs with orange, grapefruit, pineapple, and/or tomato juice. You'll help thin out mucus and ensure that your busy immune system gets enough of the vitamin C it needs to perform its defensive duties.

- Cook up some chicken soup to help clear your stuffy head. Research indicates that chicken soup is one of the most beneficial liquids you can consume when you have a cold—better than both cold and hot water—although scientists aren't exactly sure why. It may be chicken soup's ability to interfere with the body's inflammatory response or coax mucus out of the nasal passages.

- Encourage a "productive" cough by drinking hot lemonade. A productive cough is one that brings up mucus and helps to clear the airways, so it generally shouldn't be suppressed. Lemon juice acts as an expectorant, encouraging the flow of mucus to flush out viral particles. Lemon also has antimicrobial and anti-inflammatory effects. And by heating the lemonade before drinking it, you can also take advantage of the congestion-clearing power of steam. To make hot lemonade, chop up a whole lemon—rind, seeds, and all—in a blender and transfer the chopped fruit to a mug. Boil a cup of water, pour it into the mug, inhale the fragrant steam as the lemonade steeps for 5 minutes or so, add a little honey if desired, and then drink it. Help yourself to 4 or 5 cups of hot lemonade each day while you are battling a cold or the flu.

- If you're suffering from a dry, hacking cough—which is more common with the flu than with a cold—prop up your head and upper chest on pillows when you lie down.

- Soothe a harsh, dry cough with honey cough syrup. Mix together ¼ cup honey and ¼ cup apple cider vinegar. Pour the mixture into a jar or bottle and seal tightly. Shake well before using. Take 1 tablespoon every 4 hours as needed.

- Mint your own decongestant. The herb peppermint contains menthol, a common ingredient in all sorts of over-the-counter cough, cold, and flu products. And when you make a tea using peppermint, you get the congestion-clearing benefits of both the herb and the steam. You may be able to buy peppermint tea in tea bags at the grocery store or pharmacy. But you can also make your own by putting about half an ounce of peppermint leaves (from the supermarket produce section or your own garden) in a quart jar, filling the jar with boiling water, and covering it tightly. After the tea steeps for 20 minutes, strain out the leaves. Enjoy a cup right away; reheat and enjoy the remaining cups of mint tea throughout the day to help make breathing easier. If you have a fever, wrap yourself in blankets and rest in bed after you drink each cup.

- Wash away nasal inflammation with salt water. Fill a clean nasal-spray bottle with diluted salt water (1 level teaspoon salt to 4 cups lukewarm water), and squeeze the spray into each nostril 3 or 4 times. Repeat several times throughout the day as needed.

- Get temporary relief from nasal congestion with eucalyptus. Mix 1 part eucalyptus oil to 2 parts vegetable oil and smear some on the skin below your nostrils. If you can't find eucalyptus oil in a health food store or pharmacy, use a commercial vapor rub product that contains eucalyptus; check the cold and flu aisle.

- Break up congestion and make breathing a little easier by inhaling steam: Drape a towel over your head and bend over a pot of steaming-hot water, but be careful not to burn yourself. Another option, which might feel especially good just before you hop into bed, is to take a hot shower—or just run a hot shower while you sit in the closed bathroom—and inhale the moist, heated air.

- You may not feel up to this remedy if you have the flu, but if a cold has your nose all stuffed up, dig into a spicy dish made with hot peppers or topped with horseradish, both of which are known for getting the mucus flowing.

RISKY BUSINESS

Anyone can get a cold or the flu, and most people weather either one just fine. But flu and other respiratory infections can actually be quite dangerous for individuals who develop complications, such as pneumonia. Those most at risk of experiencing complications are the elderly, young children (especially those 6 months to 23 months), pregnant women, anyone with a chronic heart or lung condition or other serious disease, and those with weakened immune systems. Indeed, according to the Centers for Disease Control, the flu kills about 36,000 people in the United States each year. The deaths are primarily of the elderly and those with heart, lung, liver, or kidney disease. So if you are in a high-risk group, contact your physician at the first sign of a respiratory infection.

- An age-old remedy for the congestion of a cold or flu (or acute bronchitis) is the mustard plaster. It works mainly by increasing circulation, perspiration, and heat in the afflicted area. Its vapors may have an anti-inflammatory effect on the mucous membranes of the respiratory tract as well. To prepare a mustard plaster, mix ½ cup spicy brown mustard with 1 cup flour. Stir just enough warm water into this mixture to form a paste. Spread the paste on a cotton or muslin cloth that you've soaked in hot water and wrung out. Lay the mustard side of the plaster against your chest, cover it with a piece of dry cloth, and leave it on for 15 to 30 minutes; lift the cloth every 5 minutes to confirm that no burning or blistering is occurring. Remove the plaster promptly if it causes discomfort or extreme redness.

- Gargle with sugar water if your throat is scratchy or sore. Use 1 tablespoon corn syrup per 8 ounces of warm water, mix together well, then gargle.

- Avoid alcoholic beverages. When you're struggling with uncomfortable cold or flu symptoms, well-meaning friends and relatives may advise you to drink a hot toddy to make falling asleep easier. But alcohol is dehydrating and can increase mucous-membrane congestion, which can interfere with breathing and sleeping. And the initial sedating effect of alcohol is sometimes followed by a rebound alertness that can make falling back to sleep more difficult.

- Maintain a positive attitude. Although mind–body science is in its infancy, some researchers suggest that having an "I-can-beat-this" attitude as you fight an infection may bolster your immune function. Not all doctors agree, but staying upbeat certainly won't make the cold or flu worse.